Resistance Training

Tone Your Body For A Lifetime Of Great
Health With Resistance Training And
Resistance Band Training

Resistance Training Content

Contents

Resistance Training Introduction

Resistance – it's the impetus for growth. Without resistance we tend to stagnate, we get weak and comfortable. Resistance is what gives us challenge. It pits us against something, makes us work harder and allows us to get better.

When it comes to changing ourselves physically, resistance is the key to improvement. Resistance forces our skeletal muscles to contract. And those forceful contractions cause changes to take place within the muscle fiber. What changes? Depending on how you use that resistance it can cause you to . . .

- ✓ Build muscle
- ✓ Increase strength
- ✓ Improve endurance
- ✓ Lose fat
- ✓ Define and tone muscle

The most popular method of resistance is weight training. That's because it is a fantastic way to change your body for the better. But it is by no means the only way. Other forms of resistance training include . . .

- ✓ Resistance Bands
- ✓ Body weight
- ✓ House-hold objects
- ✓ Pulley machines

In this book you will learn to go beyond the traditional forms of resistance training in order to shape and mold your body to the way you want it. You'll be presented with a range of training routines that will, progressively, allow you to use resistance, in it's various forms, to build muscle, get stronger, shed fat and achieve a lean, athletic build.

In short, we will present you with the blueprint to use resistance to transform your body. So, get rid of any resistance you have to the idea that you can't change. Resistance is the key to the new you, and we aim to prove it.

I. Types of Resistance Training

There are three basic types of resistance movement:

(1) Isotonic
(2) Isometric
(3) Isokinetic

In this chapter, we will examine the pros of cons of each of these methods.

Isotonic Resistance

Isotonic resistance is the most familiar type of resistance exercise that we are all used to – exercising with free weights such as barbells, dumbbells or kettle-bells, as well as using our bodyweight, bands or any other equipment that allows a muscle to contract and expand against a resistance.

With isotonic resistance exercise, the weight remains constant (doesn't change) throughout the movement. The length of the muscle, however, does change. This happens as a result of concentric and eccentric contractions.

A *concentric* contraction causes shortening in muscle length. This happens when you are pushing or pulling against a resistance or weight, causing that weight to move.

An *eccentric* contraction causes lengthening in muscle length. This occurs when you return the weight to the start position of the movement. To do this effectively, you should lower the weight slowly so as to resist the effect of gravity.

The advantages of isotonic resistance training are that it is ...

✓ *Easy to do*
✓ *Easy to create overload (just add weight)*
✓ *Cheap (can be done with your own bodyweight)*

✓ *Allows you to imitate movements that are specific to sport, such as hitting a golf ball.*

The disadvantages of isotonic training are that . . .

✓ *Poor technique leads to injury*
✓ *Fatigue occurs*
✓ *To make continual advancement you need to be progressively increasing the resistance*

Isometric Resistance

Isometric resistance training involves exerting the muscles against a resistance while the length of the muscle does not actually change. As a result, there is no visible movement at the joint. This is achieved by either pushing or pulling against an immovable object.

Some bodyweight exercises that employ isometric contraction make use of what is known as sub-maximal exertion, meaning that you do not resist with full force, just enough to maintain your position. Two examples of sub-maximal exertion isometric exercise are the plank and the wall sit.

The advantages of isometric resistance are . . .

✓ It is cheap, requiring no expensive equipment
✓ It is relatively injury free
✓ It can overcome a specific muscular weakness
✓ It can be used to isolate and strengthen a weakness during a key part of an isotonic exercise, such as a third of the way through the concentric part of a barbell curl

The disadvantages of isometric resistance are . . .

✓ It develops strength at one angle only
✓ It is time consuming because you are required to contract against the resistance for a period of time

Isokinetic Resistance

Isokinetic resistance training is the newest form of resistance exercise. It allows a person to operate at a constant speed against a weight or resistance. This method uses machinery designed to develop strength through a full range of motion. The harder you push, the harder the machine pushes back. Isokinetic resistance allows for the duplication of certain sports movements, such as throwing and kicking.

The advantages of isokinetic movements are . . .

- ✓ Resistance can easily be altered (just move the weight pin)
- ✓ Develops strength through a full range of motion
- ✓ Strength is developed relatively safely

The disadvantages of isokinetic movements are . . .

- ✓ Machines are expensive
- ✓ Does not develop ligament and tendon strength as much as isotonic training because the machine provides the stability of the resistance

Building Your Routine

When structuring your individual workout program you need to use a combination of all three resistance types in order to achieve maximum benefit. The majority of your workout, however, should be built around isotonic exercises. The reason is simple . . .

Isotonic exercises do the best job of working all of your muscles through a full range of motion.

Take an exercise like the dumbbell bench press, for example. The very act of getting the dumbbells into position as you lay down on the bench involves a whole host of small synergistic muscle groups. Doing the bench press on an isokinetic machine doesn't allow for stimulation of these muscles. Then, as you press the weight up and then slowly descend you are working the target muscle group (pectorals) through a full range of motion, involving both concentric (up) and eccentric (down) pathways. This does not occur with an isometric exercise, which limits the effect to a single angle.

There is still a place for both isometric and isokinetic movements in an effective routine, however. Such moves as the plank and wall sit are very effective at developing strength in the abdominals and quads, respectively. They will also allow you to overcome a strength plateau on a specific exercise when you perform 30 second static holds at the sticking point of the exercise. Machines, that utilise isokinetic resistance are generally best for beginners as they get used to the proper form of a movement. Once they have mastered it, they should then go on to free weight isotonic moves.

II. Weight Resistance Training

Why Weights?

Weight training has been and is being used by people all over this planet to create their ideal body. And we're not just referring to bodybuilders here. We're talking regular people who want to lose kilos, firm problem areas and produce some definition on their bodies. But not only that . . .

The benefits of weight training start on the inside and radiate outwards. After your first workout you'll notice an immediate improvement in your self esteem. Your mental outlook will brighten. You will develop the vital qualities of success - self discipline, focus, goal setting and resilience. Your new inner strength will begin to be reflected in how you project yourself - your posture will improve, you'll be looking people in the eye more readily and you'll be able to make decisions about your health more decisively.
In addition, weight training will provide you with the following benefits . . .

- ✓ Increased strength and endurance
- ✓ Improved sleep
  Reduced stress
- ✓ Stronger bones
- ✓ More muscle
- ✓ Boosted metabolism to burn off energy and, therefore, fat

Weight Resistance Training Reps and Sets

The number of repetitions (reps) you perform goes a long way toward determining the effect of your training. More than exercise selection, rep count will affect whether the workout primarily builds muscle, enhances strength or burns off fat. The following guidelines will help you to determine the rep range for your chosen outcome . . .

For maximum strength use a very heavy weight that allows no more than 2-6 reps.

For muscle mass use a rep range of between 6-12 reps.

For a fat burn focus, use a rep range of between 8 and 15 reps.

The number of reps you are able to perform is directly related to the amount of weight you can lift. A person who is using a rep range of 4-6 will, therefore, be using a much heavier weight than the person who is doing the same exercise for a 15 rep count. Regardless of the rep count, however, the last repetition of a movement should always be the last rep you could have performed with that weight and with good form. If it isn't, then you need to increase the resistance.

A set is made up of a number of repetitions performed without any rest. There is a vast amount of variation in the number of sets that people perform, again depending on the specific training goal. In the workouts to follow we will be using a range of set protocols.

Rest between sets is a crucial factor in determining the effectiveness of your program. For endurance and fat loss, you should take minimal rest periods of no more than 30 seconds. For those intent on building muscle, rest periods should typically be between 90 and 120 seconds. When power is your goal, you should give yourself between 3 and 5 minutes to fully recover from a set before going into the next set.

How to Design an Efficient Routine

Know the End Goal

The magazines and websites are loaded with the training routines of the latest A-List athlete or movie stars. The gist of all of these stories is that if you follow their routine, you'll end up looking just like them. That is a load of rubbish! Those people are on a different planet to most of us. They have the luxury of training for three hours each day, hiring a personal trainer *and* a chef to prepare all of their meals. So, forget about what anyone else is doing and consider why you are doing what you are doing.

Your training goal needs to be at the fore-front of your mind, because it will determine how you train.

Do you primarily want to improve your health? If so, you don't need to get down and dirty with the heavy-ass weights. Moderate intensity sets of 8-15 reps will be more than sufficient.

Do you want to overhaul the physical look of your body by adding lean muscle tissue? You need to perform 3 sets per muscle group, splitting your sessions into body part workouts and getting heavy in the 6-12 rep range.

If you are working with weights to train for an athletic event then your workouts will be different again. You should tailor your weight training to the specific event. For a hilly 10 k run, you need to give more attention to your quads and glutes, for instance.

Order Your Exercises Correctly

You should always begin training by working your larger muscle groups and finishing with your smaller ones. That's because your smaller muscles, such as the biceps, are linking muscles that connect the weight to your larger muscles groups. If they are already exhausted by the time you get to training them, then the large muscle group isn't going to get a very effective workout.

Your upper body should be trained as follows . . .

- o Chest and Back (either first)
- o Shoulders
- o Biceps and Triceps (either first)
- o Forearms

Your lower body should be trained as follows . . .

- o Glutes
- o Thighs
- o Hamstrings
- o Calves

Selecting the Weight

As already mentioned, the weight you select will be directly proportional to the number of reps you will be performing. The following chart gives a good indication of the percentage of your one rep maximum that you should be lifting on a range of rep counts.

Number of Reps	%age of One Rep Max
1	100
2-3	95
4-5	90
6-7	85
8-9	80
10-11	75
12-13	70
14-15	65
16-20	60

Build Around Compound Movements

There are many exercise options for each body part. Some rely heavily on synergists and stabilizers. Most of these are compound movements such as bench press, seated rows and squats. Others rely only moderately on synergists and stabilizers. These are more focused exercises like triceps kick-backs and leg extensions.

Compound movements duplicate the ways that you use muscles in everyday life. Think about it - when was the last time you did a motion resembling a tricep kick-back outside of the gym? In contrast, every time you push open a door, or help a neighbor to move a couch or refrigerator, what you are doing looks a whole lot like a bench press. Every time you lift a heavy box from the floor, the motion resembles a squat. And if you have to put that box on a top shelf, you are essentially doing a military press.

The kind of functional strength resulting from major body exercises is much more important in terms of health and effectiveness in day-to-day physical activity than the limited, specific strength resulting from isolation exercises. Major body compound exercises are also far more effective at burning fat.

Fat Burning Movements

Forget about the treadmill and the Elliptical machine. Going hard on compound movements burns a ton of calories. Yes, calories. Most people don't actually realize the energy it takes to get under a squat rack and bend up and down a dozen times with a sizable weight across your trapezius. Focusing on compound exercises such as squats, lunges, rows, presses and dead-lifts will have you puffing like a locomotive.

Using compound movements as the foundation of your weight training routine will also give your body a huge metabolic lift. In fact, it boosts your rate of calorie burning (metabolism) for hours after the workout is over. This is due to a phenomena known as post exercise oxygen consumption (EPOC). This means that compound training will allow you to burn extra calories even while you're watching TV. In addition, there is a high energy cost in repairing damaged muscle cells as a result of your workouts. And any muscle that you build requires more calories to maintain.

Heart Health Movement

Another benefit of compound movements is that they will improve your cardiovascular fitness. Compound movements like squats and dead-lifts will shunt the blood around your whole body. Your heart and lungs will be more efficient and you will be dramatically reducing your susceptibility to a host of cardiovascular diseases.

Top 4 Compound Movements to Burn Fat Fast

Squats

Position yourself under the bar and lift it off the rack. Step back and stand with your feet spread slightly wider than shoulder width and pointing slightly outward. Keep your back straight, your chest thrust out and your head up. Now tense your abdominal wall, bend you knees and lower your body until your thighs are parallel with the floor. To avoid excess strain on the knees, don't go down any further. While squatting, keep your head up and your back slightly arched.

Deadlifts

Load a barbell and set it on the floor. Squat in front of it with your feet shoulder width apart. Grab it overhead with your hands just outside your legs, your shoulders over or just behind the bar, your arms straight and your back flat or slightly arched.

Simple as it sounds, all you really do is stand up. The key is to push with your heels and pull the weight to your body as you stand. Pause with the weight, but don't lean back, then slowly return to the starting position. Pause with the weight on the floor and reset your body over the bar. You defeat the purpose of the dead-lift if you use momentum to knock out the reps.

Renegade Row

Lie on the floor with a pair of dumbbells positioned beneath your armpits. Grab the dumbbells and support yourself as if you were about to begin a push up. Keeping your body in a straight line (don't bend at the waist), row one of the dumbbells up to your lats. Repeat on the other side to complete one rep,

Lunges

Stand shoulder width part, with a dumbbell in each hand at your sides. Keeping your back arched, take an exaggerated step forward with your right leg. Lower your rear leg until that knee just touches the floor. Now reverse the movement to return to the start position. Repeat with the other leg for one rep.

III. Sample Weight Routines

Total Body Fat Loss Workout

Follow this 16 exercise no-rest program to give your body a total work-out, both inside and out. Perform just one set of each exercise. Aerobic exercises last for 1 minute. Give yourself a maximum of 15 seconds to get to the next exercise.

(1) Squats
(2) Treadmill
(3) Lat Pull-downs
(4) Skipping
(5) Bench Press
(6) Cycle
(7) Seated Shoulder Press with Dumb-bells
(8) Stepper
(9) Barbell Bench Press
(10)   Mini trampoline sprints
(11)   Tricep Pushdowns
(12)   Treadmill
(13)   Standing Calf Raises
(14)   Skipping
(15)   Leg Extensions
(16)   Cycle

If you're planning to hit the gym every lunch-time, do the above program on Monday, Wednesday and Friday. On Tuesday and Thursday, focus exclusively on burning fat and improving your cardiovascular fitness and recovery time by devoting your time to the treadmill. Set the timer for 24 minutes. After a two minute warm-up, sprint at maximum speed for 60 seconds. Then, take your feet off the running track for a 30 second recovery. Continue this routine until your timer shows 2 minutes remaining. Finish with a slow warm down.

Muscle Building Compound Workout

The bodybuilding magazines and websites have made building muscle extremely complicated (and extremely lucrative) to the extent that every guy thinks he needs to do at least 6 exercise for his biceps and triceps alone. Split routines are the default workout style. Anything less is for the pencil neck geek and the clueless klutz.

Let everyone else in the gym carry on their merry multi exercise, isolation focused way. You are going to train smarter. For a hard gainer to build muscle what's needed is increasing the weights, dropping the reps, taking longer rest periods between sets and to focus on the basic compound exercises. That's why your entire routine is going to consist of the big 6 mass builders . . .

Squats

Dead-lifts

Pull Ups

Bench Press

Military Press

That's it! No barbell curls, no pec dec flyes, no lying leg curls. Put all of your energy and focus into the compound exercises that are already working every muscle in your body.

What's more, you'll only be in the gym twice a week. Go with Monday and Thursday, to provide maximum rest between workouts. Do not be tempted to do more exercise than this - it will be counterproductive. Just make sure that every single second of every workout is full on.

From now on, your training mindset needs to be: ***Get in, work your body like hell, then get out.***

Unless you get your choice of exercise right, you're going to be wasting a lot of time in the gym for very little reward. Heavy compound movements are the key to building muscle mass. These are the multi-joint movements that work a variety of muscle groups simultaneously. They also simulate real life movements, like squatting down or lifting something off the floor. Prime examples of compound movements are chin ups, squats and the bench press. These exercises are not only the best way to build bulk and they will get you stronger quicker than anything else. And, because they work muscle groups simultaneously, they are far more time efficient than isolation movements.

The following exercises will form the basis of your training:

Squats

Dead-lifts

Pull Ups

Bench Press

Military Press

Perform 4 sets of each movement on a pyramid rep / set scheme as follows

Set One – 12 reps

Set Two – 10 reps

Set Three – 8 reps

Set Four 6 reps

As the reps decrease in each succeeding set, increase the weight in accordance with the chart on Page 11. You should give yourself between 60-90 seconds rest between sets.

IV. Bodyweight Resistance Training

As long as gravity exists, your own bodyweight can provide a vigorous home workout that does all the good things that any weights based routine does - that is build muscle and promote fat loss. That means that you don't have to spend a small fortune to get fit. Travel is never a problem because you are always carrying your workout equipment - your body - with you. A hotel room or a friend's house is as good a location as your own home.

One unique benefit of no-equipment exercises is that they make it much more convenient to take advantage of a valuable workout technique called circuit training. In circuits, you do one set of each exercise in the routine before doing a second set of any exercise. Moving quickly from exercise to exercise allows you to the more work done in less time - and this is an even more efficient process when there's no weight to adjust or station to set up. Circuit training is also a fantastic way to enhance the fat loss effects of resistance training. It boosts your metabolism to burn calories like crazy - all the while, allowing you to build, shape and define every muscle group in your body.

Bodyweight Circuit

Start with 5 to 10 minutes of continuous activity that involves large muscle groups - such as doing jumping jacks, running up stairs or skipping. Then do each exercise on your circuit list in succession, pausing only long enough to get ready for the next one. Start with 12 repetitions of each exercise, eventually working your way up to 20. Go through the circuit twice.

The Circuit

Push Ups: Set yourself on the ground, face down with your hands slightly wider than shoulder width apart. Your feet should be touching. Keeping your body in a straight line, rise up so that your arms are fully extended. Tense your buttocks and tighten your abs to prevent your butt from lifting you into a 'v' position. Look straight ahead rather than down. Now steadily lower yourself until your elbows are at a 90-degree angle. When your chest touches the floor, explode back up to the start position.

Modified Pull Ups: Set up a bar or equivalent between two uprights so that it is positioned horizontally at waist height. Grasp the bar with an overhand grip and lower yourself so that you are hanging underneath it with feet extended out. Now, with your back arched, pull up so that your chin touches the bar. Lower to full extension and repeat.

Reverse Dips: Position yourself in front of a low bench facing away with your hands behind you resting on the bench. Your hands should be about 6 inches apart and your legs extended in front of you so that your body forms a straight line. From this position, bend at the elbows to lower your core area towards the floor. From a bottom position power back up, focusing on your triceps to do the work.

Squats: Start with your feet shoulders width apart and ensure your back is arched. Hold your hands out directly in front of you palms, parallel to the ground (you can add weight as you progress by holding a book in your outstretched hands throughout the movement). Slowly bend your knees and lower your body until your thighs are parallel with the ground. Keep your back straight and avoid bending throughout the movement. Don't worry if you can't get your thighs lower than parallel to the ground to start. This can be your goal over time. Don't sacrifice a straight back and good posture by trying to go too low too soon.

Box Jumps: Start with your feet shoulder width apart and the box about a foot in front of you. Bend your knees into a semi-squat position, trail your hands back behind your waist and throw them forward as you leap up onto the box. You'll roll forward onto the balls of your feet as you spring up for your leap. Imagine you're trying to jump across a small stream from a standing start using both feet at the same time. Both feet must leave the ground and land flat on the box at the same time (try to avoid landing with just the balls of your feet).

Mason Crunches: Mason Twists: Sit with your back arched and knees slightly bent. Your feet should be just off the floor. Now grasp your hands together in front of your knees. Use a twisting motion to touch your hands to the floor on either side of you in a fast paced motion. Be sure to make solid contact on each side and keep your feet up throughout. Both sides count as one rep.

Jumping Split Lunges: Standing, feet together, and with hands on hips, bend your knees and jump up, landing with your right foot in front of you and your left foot behind. You'll want to get as deep a bend in your knees as possible

Mountain Climbers: Start in a traditional push-up position, keeping your core tight. Bring one knee up as close to your chest as possible while balancing on the opposite foot, and then quickly switch legs. Keep your butt down and your palms on the floor at all times

The above circuit routine will allow you to work every major muscle group of your body, while torching body fat, revving up your metabolism and improving the efficiency of your heart and lungs. Do this work-out every second day. On your off days, do some High Intensity Interval Training (HIIT). The combination of circuit training and HIIT will take your fat burning efforts to the next level, allowing you to hone in on that fit, athletic, fat free fee body that so many desire but so few achieve.

V. Resistance Band Training

Rubber bands provide a resistance workout at a fraction of the cost of free weights and machines. They won't make you as strong as free weights will, but they will challenge your muscles in a unique way and are effective in achieving a degree of muscle and strength gain as well as fat loss when performed as part of a circuit. Because they don't rely on gravity or weight for their resistance, bands provide resistance during both the concentric and eccentric part of the movement. This is a distinct advantage over other resistance options, which offer little in the way of eccentric resistance.

Another distinct advantage of resistance bands is their light weight and portability. You can easily slip them into your workout bag (try doing that with a pair of dumbbells. That makes them a great option when you're traveling or just can't get to the gym.

Using Bands Efficiently For Maximum Results

You can purchase bands for next to nothing. If you want to splurge, get bands with plastic handle attachments. This will make it easier to do such exercises as bicep curls. Generally the shorter and thicker than band, the harder it is to pull and the more resistance it provides. Some manufacturers, such as *Life Line,* produce bands in different colors to represent the relative resistance levels.

When using bands it is very important that you follow some basic safety precautions . . .

o Make sure that the band is securely in place before you start your set. If you have to hook your foot over the band, make sure that it is under the midsole area.
o If you have to hold the bands in your hands, loop the ends around your palms – make sure, though, that it doesn't cut off your circulation.

The following band fitness circuit will give you an effective total body workout and can be done anywhere, any time. Perform 8-15 reps on each exercise, doing the exercises with no rest between them. Rest for 90 seconds and then repeat. Work up to doing 4 rounds of the circuit.

Band Squat

o Hold the end of a band in each hand and stand on top of the centre of the band so that your feet are hip-width apart and your hands are at your sides. Stand tall with your abdominals pulled in and shoulders squeezed.
o Sit back and down, as if you're sitting in a chair. Bend you knees and lower yourself as far as you can without leaning your upper body more than a few inches forward. Never go below parallel to the floor and don't allow your knees to move out in front of your toes.
o Push up through your heels to drive back to the start position. Keep your head up and eyes focused directly in front of you throughout.

Band Hamstring Stretch

o Lie down on the floor with your feet flat on the floor and your knees bent, with your arms to your sides.
o Bring your right foot toward your chest and wrap an exercise band around the arch of your foot. Exhale as you extend your right leg toward the ceiling. Repeat on the other side

Band Lat Pulldown

- Sit in a chair with your feet hip width apart and hold an end of the exercise band in each hand. Raise your arms over your head with your left palm facing in and your right palm facing forward just above shoulder level. Your elbows should be slightly bent. Stand tall with your abdominals pulled in and your knees relaxed.
- Keep your left arm still. Bend your right elbow down and out to the side, as if you're shooting an arrow straight up into the air. Keeping your wrist straight, pull the band until your right hand is to the side of your right shoulder, the band is tight, and your right elbow points down. Slowly straighten your arm. Switch sides, alternating as you complete the set.

Band External Rotation

- Tie a band around a stable object. Stand with your left side toward the tied off end of the band. Hold the other end of the band in your right hand with your palm facing in. Bend your elbow 90 degrees.
- Keeping your elbow in place, move your hand a few inches away from you to increase tension in the band, then slowly move it back to the start position. After you've completed a set with your right arm, turn around and do an equal number of reps with your left arm.

Band Shoulder Stretch

- Stand up tall, feet about shoulder width apart, holding both ends of the band in front of your thighs.

o Inhale as you straighten your arms and raise them overhead. As you exhale, move your arms further behind your head, but don't arch your back.

Band Triceps Extension

- o While holding onto one end of the band with your left hand, stand with your feet as wide as your hips and place your left palm over the front of your shoulder. Hold the other end of the band in your right hand with your palm facing inward.
- o Bend your right elbow so that it's at waist height and pointing behind you. You can lean slightly forward from your hips if you find the position comfortable, but always keep your abs in and your knees relaxed.
- o Keeping your elbows stationary, straighten your arm out behind you so the band gets tighter as you go, but don't allow your elbow to lock. Then bend your elbow so your hand travels back to your waist. Reposition the band to work your left triceps.

VI. Resistance Training Forever

Developing resistance training as a lifestyle habit is one of the wisest things that you can do in life. It will keep you running smoothly on the inside while looking fantastic on the outside. To ensure that you are making the most of your resistance workouts, here are some key principles to train by . . .

(1) **Add Weight:** If you are training regularly, supplementing wisely and getting enough rest, you will be getting stronger by the week. To keep placing stress on your muscles you have got to increase the load on them. If you don't, your muscles will adapt to the load and have no reason to keep responding. You don't have to add a 20-pound plate every workout but you can and should be able to slip on an extra pound or two. Make sure that you don't sacrifice perfect form for the extra weight and keep your rep rate at 2 seconds up and 4 seconds down.

(2) **Decrease Rest:** In the gym, stress on your muscles is a good thing - in fact it's the whole point of what you're doing. When you do a set, your muscle stress level skyrockets. Then when you rest the stress begins dropping back. Rest long enough and your stress level will be back to zero. Then on the next set it will get back to where it was during the first set - and then drop back during the next rest period. But what happens when you shorten the rest period? Your body doesn't have enough time for the stress to level to drop back completely, so you'll end up with a stair step effect. The intensity threshold will be cumulatively increasing with every set. Your work out will be far more effective. Try reducing your rest period to just 30 seconds per set. Initially the challenge will be to keep the weights from slipping back. Then once your body adjusts to the reduced rest time, you'll be able to start adding weight again.

(3) **Add Reps:** From week to week, as your body gets stronger, you will find it less stressful to meet your rep range. When that happens you should add reps. If, for instance, you have been doing 8 reps per set on barbell curls, add a rep or two each workout until you are comfortably able to hit 12. Then it's time to increase the weight by a couple of pounds and take it back to 8 reps.

On lower body exercises, such as squats and let extensions, keep your rep progressions between 10 and 15. Once you hit 15, drop back to 10 and add some weight to the bar.

VII. Wrap Up

When it comes to resistance training, if you're not moving forward then you're standing still. And if you're standing still, you're not making progress. Never go into a workout intent on doing the same as you did last time. Set a goal before you even pull into the parking lot to make your workout harder by lifting more weight, doing more reps or reducing your rest time. That way you'll be making real, meaningful progress towards your goals - and making the most of your resistance training.

Sage Surefire

Subscribe to our list to get notified of new book releases from Sage Surefire. We notify you of new book releases, updates to the books, and when a book is given away free.

Click here to subscribe

You'll like my other books.

Women Bodybuilding: Build a lean, sexy, toned, curvy body without getting bulky

http://www.amazon.com/gp/product/B00YB9SAN0?*Version*=1&*entries*=0

CrossFit Training: Build a lean, athletic, sexy body with fresh and exciting crossfit workouts

http://www.amazon.com/gp/product/B00Z14BENW?*Version*=1&*entries*=0

Building Muscle: Bullshit free secrets to building muscle

http://www.amazon.com/gp/product/B010INJBPS?*Version*=1&*entries*=0

HIIT Workouts: Get HIIT fit, fast-track your way to a shredded, super-fit new you

http://www.amazon.com/gp/product/B010MSYK96?*Version*=1&*entries*=0

Absolute Fitness Kettlebell Workouts

http://www.amazon.com/gp/product/B010Z9TJDO